21ST Century Skills INNOVATION LIBRARY

Exploring the Internet of Things

Smart Healthcare

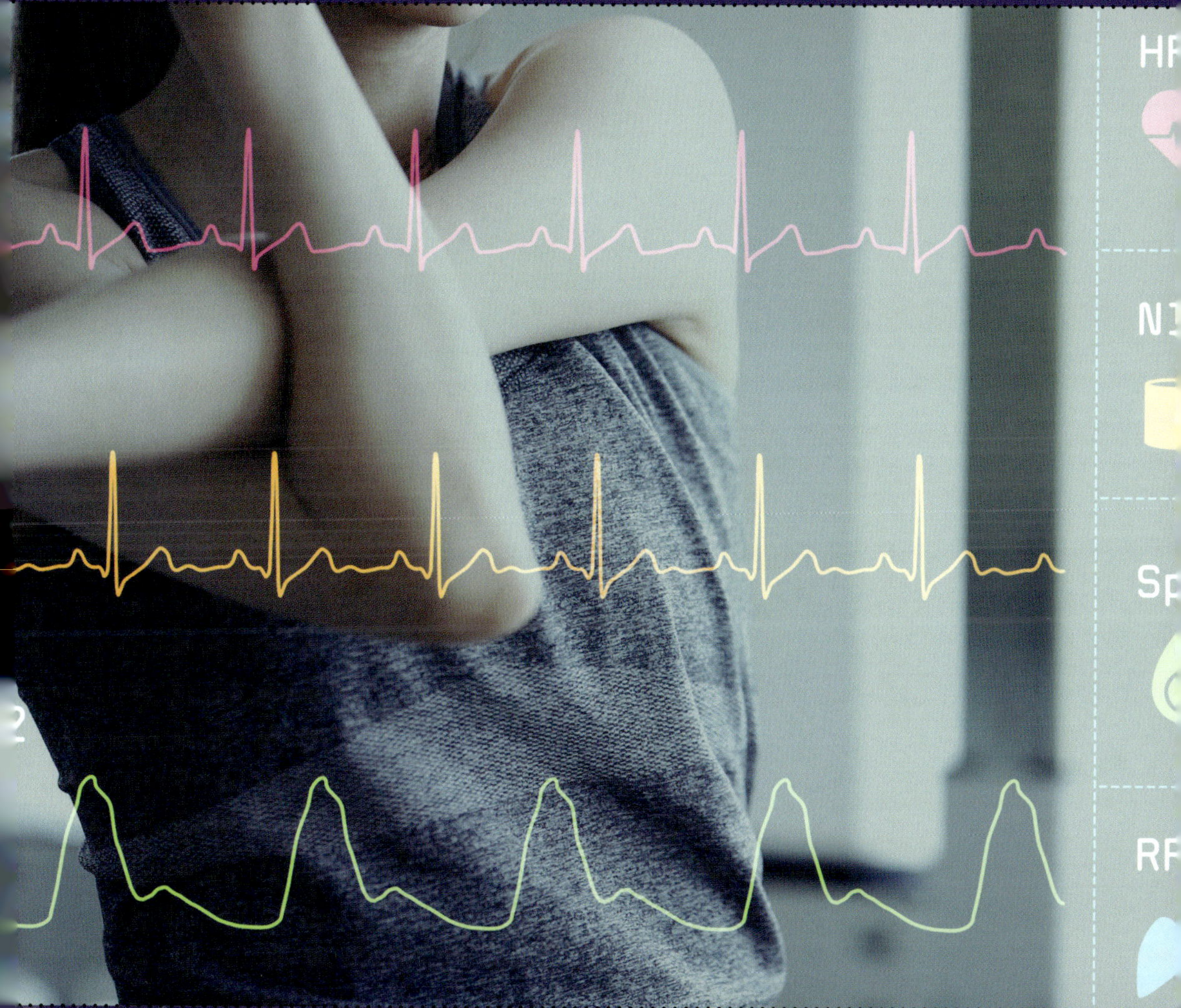

Martin Gitlin

Cherry Lake Press

Published in the United States of America by Cherry Lake Publishing
Ann Arbor, Michigan
www.cherrylakepublishing.com

Reading Adviser: Marla Conn, MS, Ed., Literacy specialist, Read-Ability, Inc.

Photo Credits: © metamorworks/Shutterstock, cover, 1, 23; © fizkes/Shutterstock, 5; © Photographee.eu/Shutterstock, 7; © Juhan Sonin/Flickr, 8; © Wavebreakmedia Ltd/Dreamstime.com, 9; © Vershinin89/Shutterstock, 10; © David Bleeker Photography/Alamy Stock Photo, 13; © Rob Marmion/Shutterstock, 15; © sutadimage/Shutterstock, 16; © Gorodenkoff/Shutterstock, 17; © Monkey Business Images/Shutterstock, 18, 24; © Airman 1st Class Bailee Darbasie/U.S. Air Force, 21; © TZIDO SUN/Shutterstock, 27; © Stepan Kapl/Shutterstock, 29

Graphic Element Credits: © Ohn Mar/Shutterstock.com, back cover, multiple interior pages;
© Dmitrieva Katerina/Shutterstock.com, back cover, multiple interior pages;
© advent/Shutterstock.com, back cover, front cover, multiple interior pages;
© Visual Generation/Shutterstock.com, multiple interior pages;
© anfisa focusova/Shutterstock.com, front cover, multiple interior pages;
© Babich Alexander/Shutterstock.com, back cover, front cover, multiple interior pages

Library of Congress Cataloging-in-Publication Data has been filed and is available at catalog.loc.gov.

Names: Gitlin, Marty, author.
Title: Smart healthcare / by Martin Gitlin.
Description: Ann Arbor, Michigan : Cherry Lake Publishing, 2020. | Series: Exploring the internet of things | Includes index.
Identifiers: LCCN 2020003068 (print) | LCCN 2020003069 (ebook) | ISBN 9781534168947 (hardcover) | ISBN 9781534170629 (paperback) | ISBN 9781534172463 (pdf) | ISBN 9781534174306 (ebook)
Subjects: LCSH: Medical informatics. | Medical technology.
Classification: LCC R858 .G537 2020 (print) | LCC R858 (ebook) | DDC 610.285–dc23
LC record available at https://lccn.loc.gov/2020003068
LC ebook record available at https://lccn.loc.gov/2020003069

Printed in the United States of America
Corporate Graphics

Table of Contents

Introduction

The process has remained the same for decades. People feel sick. They often do not know their exact illness. So they visit a doctor or take a trip to the hospital. Sometimes the problem is severe. There is no time for an appointment. The patient heads right to the emergency room.

The relationship between doctors and patients has been limited to exams and phone calls. Some interactions in recent years have included emails and text messages. It is a system that has worked. But it can be better. And the Internet of Things (IoT) has helped create positive changes.

IoT **sensors** connect devices to the internet and to each other. **Data** is delivered to doctors through these objects in real time.

For example, a company called Spry Health has created smart wristbands for people suffering from chronic illness. The health data collected by the smart wearable device is sent

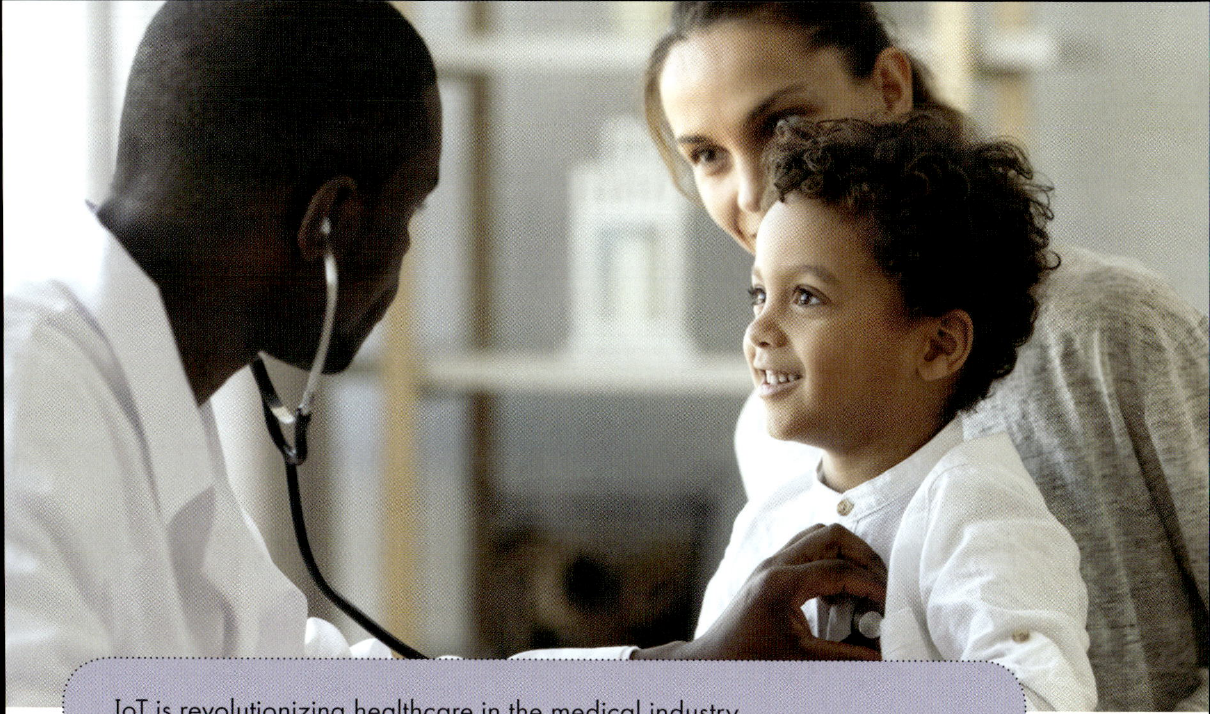

IoT is revolutionizing healthcare in the medical industry.

directly to a team of healthcare professionals. People can rest easy knowing their health is being closely **monitored**.

IoT in healthcare connects doctors with patients remotely. It allows doctors and hospitals to monitor patient health in real time. They can **diagnose** problems without seeing patients. They can suggest treatments and **prescribe** medicines. The result is an easier patient-doctor relationship. Limiting unnecessary medical visits allows doctors to pay more attention to the patients they need to see face-to-face.

The data delivered by IoT has impacted quality and ease of healthcare. Time saved and speed in which a diagnosis can be made can have a huge effect. IoT technology impacts doctors, patients, families, and hospitals.

CHAPTER ONE

Smart Medical Devices

The Internet of Things creates stronger links between patient and doctor. A new era began with wearable activity trackers. IoT wearables such as Fitbit promote good health. They monitor blood pressure and heart rate. Devices have since become more advanced. They measure a wider range of health issues. And the data they provide can be shared with doctors.

The most troubling disease in the modern era is cancer. Scientists have worked in vain for years to find a cure. But a smart monitoring system using a connected weight scale and blood pressure cuff track cancer **symptoms**. They also update doctors on how well treatments are working.

Diabetes is another widespread disease. It is defined by elevated levels of blood sugar. People with diabetes must take **insulin** to raise their energy level. They must also monitor their blood sugar levels constantly. IoT technology has a solution. A sensor placed under the skin reads blood sugar levels. It sends

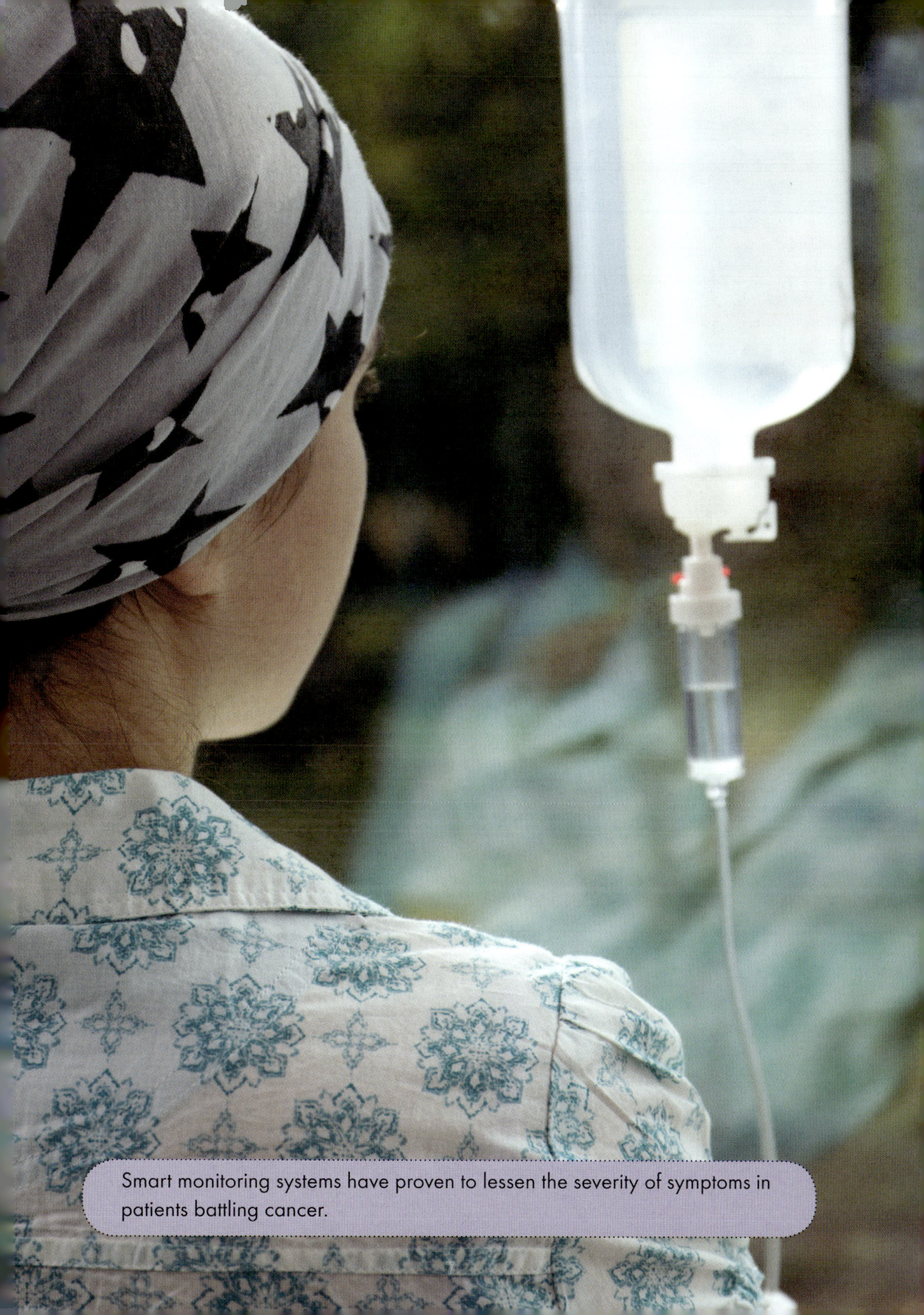

Smart monitoring systems have proven to lessen the severity of symptoms in patients battling cancer.

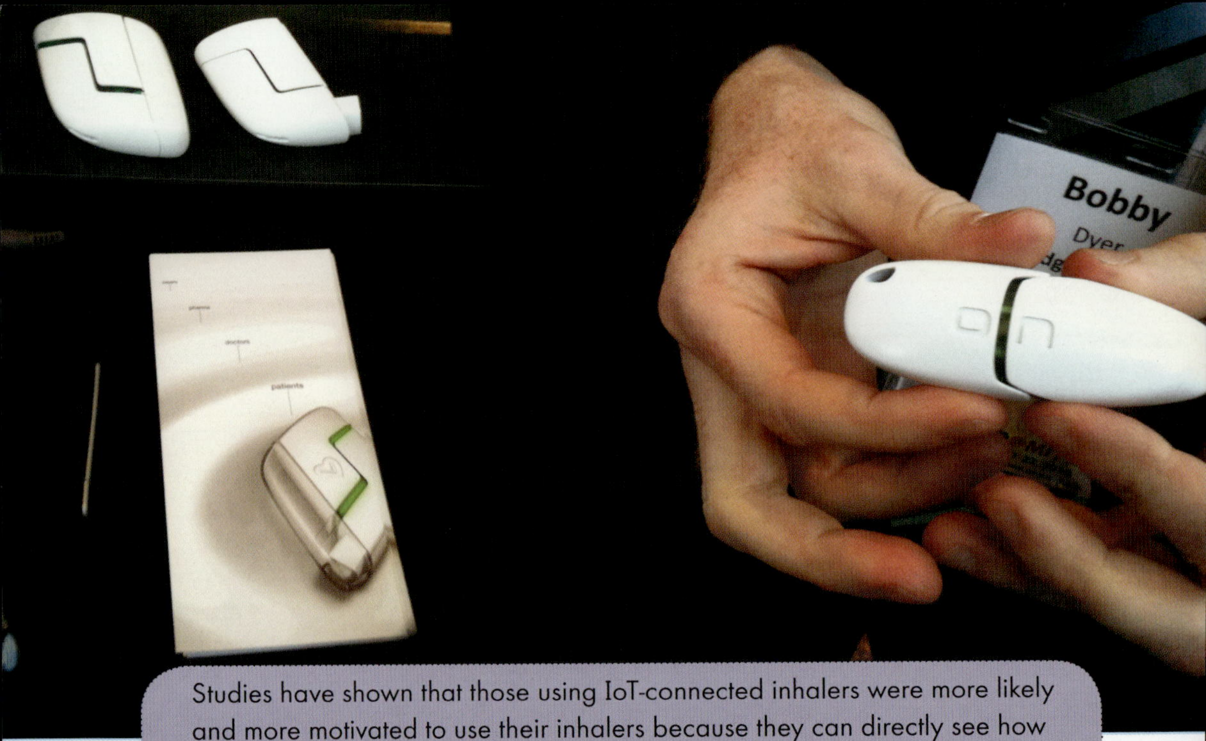

Studies have shown that those using IoT-connected inhalers were more likely and more motivated to use their inhalers because they can directly see how it improves their health via an app.

data to mobile apps. Wearers easily check information and trends. The information is then received by medical professionals.

Asthma patients can also be helped by IoT. A smart inhaler provides insight on what is causing a patient's symptoms. It tracks use of medications. It even predicts levels of **allergens** in the air that prevent clear breathing. One smart wearable monitor provides an immediate warning of an asthma attack. The smart device detects symptoms before it strikes. It vibrates to warn the victim. It lets caregivers know an attack is coming. And it can even send medication reminders.

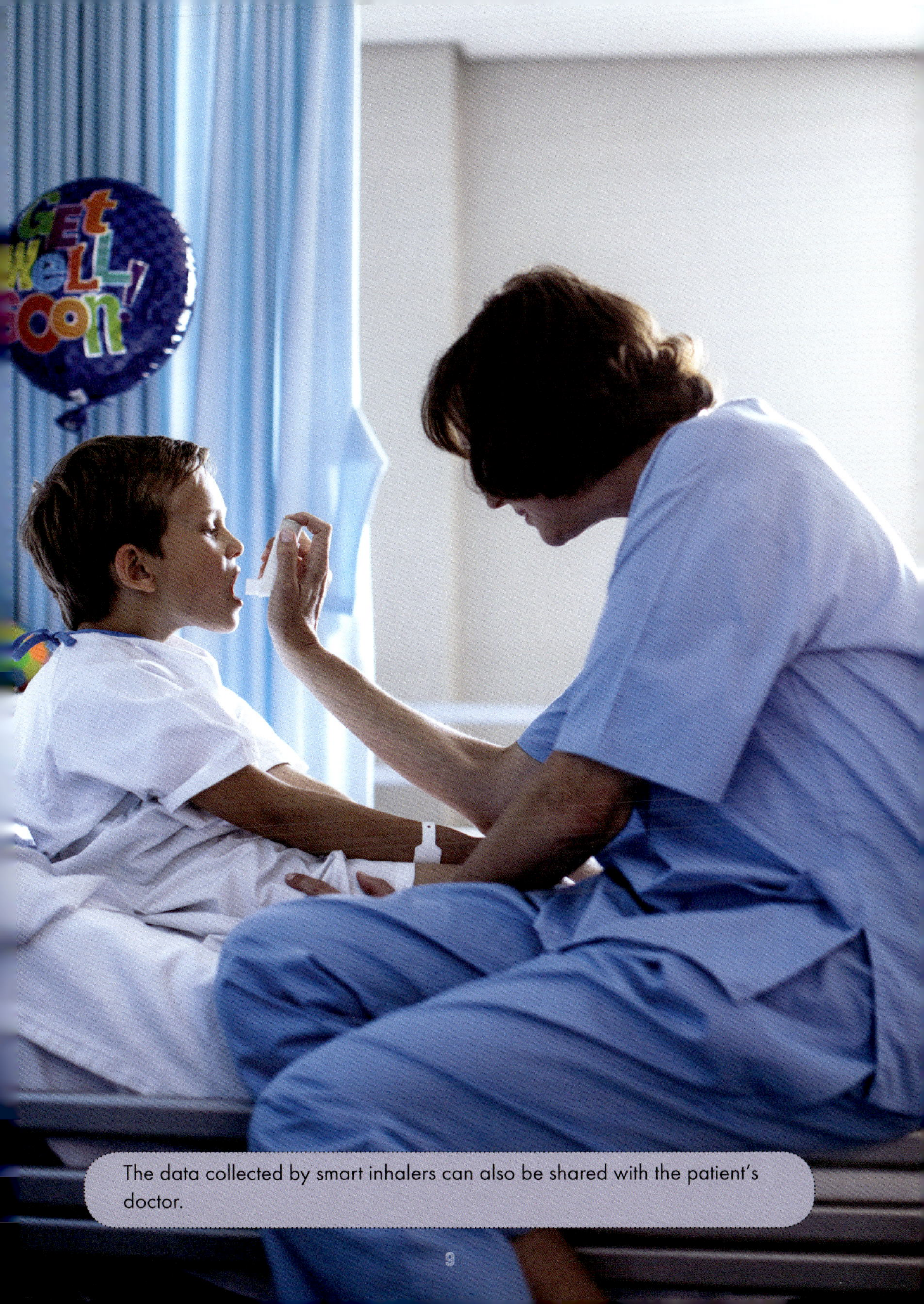

The data collected by smart inhalers can also be shared with the patient's doctor.

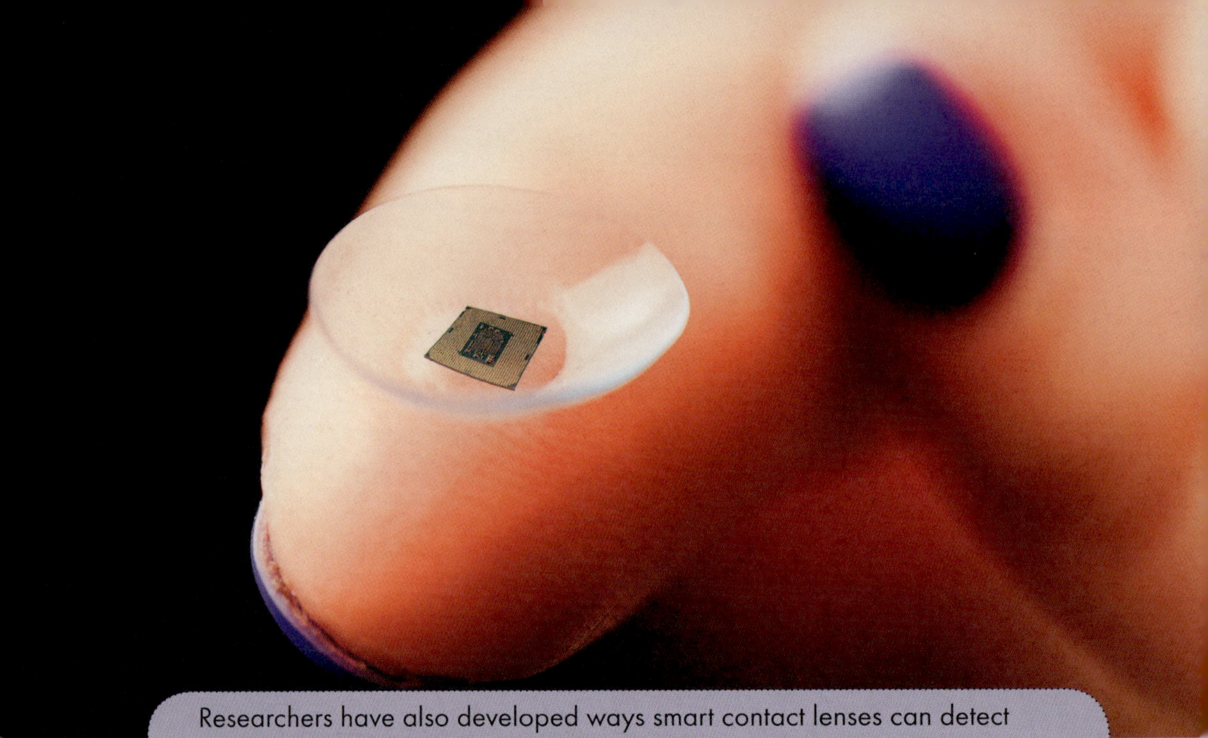

Researchers have also developed ways smart contact lenses can detect early symptoms of glaucoma.

There are even smart devices that you can eat! Researchers have created an edible medical device that can help doctors better measure and monitor the inside of a person's stomach. This could help diagnose a multitude of disorders and diseases, including **gastroparesis**. One example of this is the SmartPill®.

Another intriguing IoT device is the smart contact lens. About 250 million people suffer from forms of visual impairment, including **cataracts**. Lenses with a wireless cup and tiny sensors could treat such conditions. The potential of smart contact lenses extends beyond eye health. They could also tell people with diabetes that their blood sugar level has dropped. And they could alert doctors of dangerous changes in condition.

IoT technology does not only monitor physical issues. One Apple Watch app assesses patients with depression. The wearable monitors mood and awareness. A study showed it to be as reliable as traditional **cognitive** testing.

The **influx** of IoT devices will continue to impact healthcare. But are there any drawbacks?

THE BATTLE AGAINST PARKINSON'S

Parkinson's disease is a terrible illness. It affects the central nervous system. It causes tremors that negatively impact movement. Parkinson's often worsens and can result in death. Doctors have prescribed treatment and medications. But they cannot personalize an approach for each individual. They cannot monitor every movement.

IoT technology is changing that. Sensors placed inside the body can track how effectively drugs are working. That allows doctors to devise and revise plans to improve treatment.

Connected devices can also be worn. Or they can be embedded in spots around the home. One can be placed on a refrigerator door. It notes issues associated with Parkinson's. It can detect if a person grabs the handle differently or struggles to open the door.

There is no downtime for such sensors. They can monitor movements 24 hours a day. They even monitor how the disease is affecting sleep patterns.

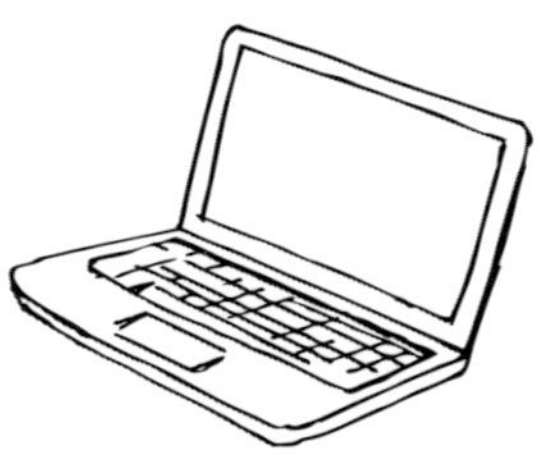

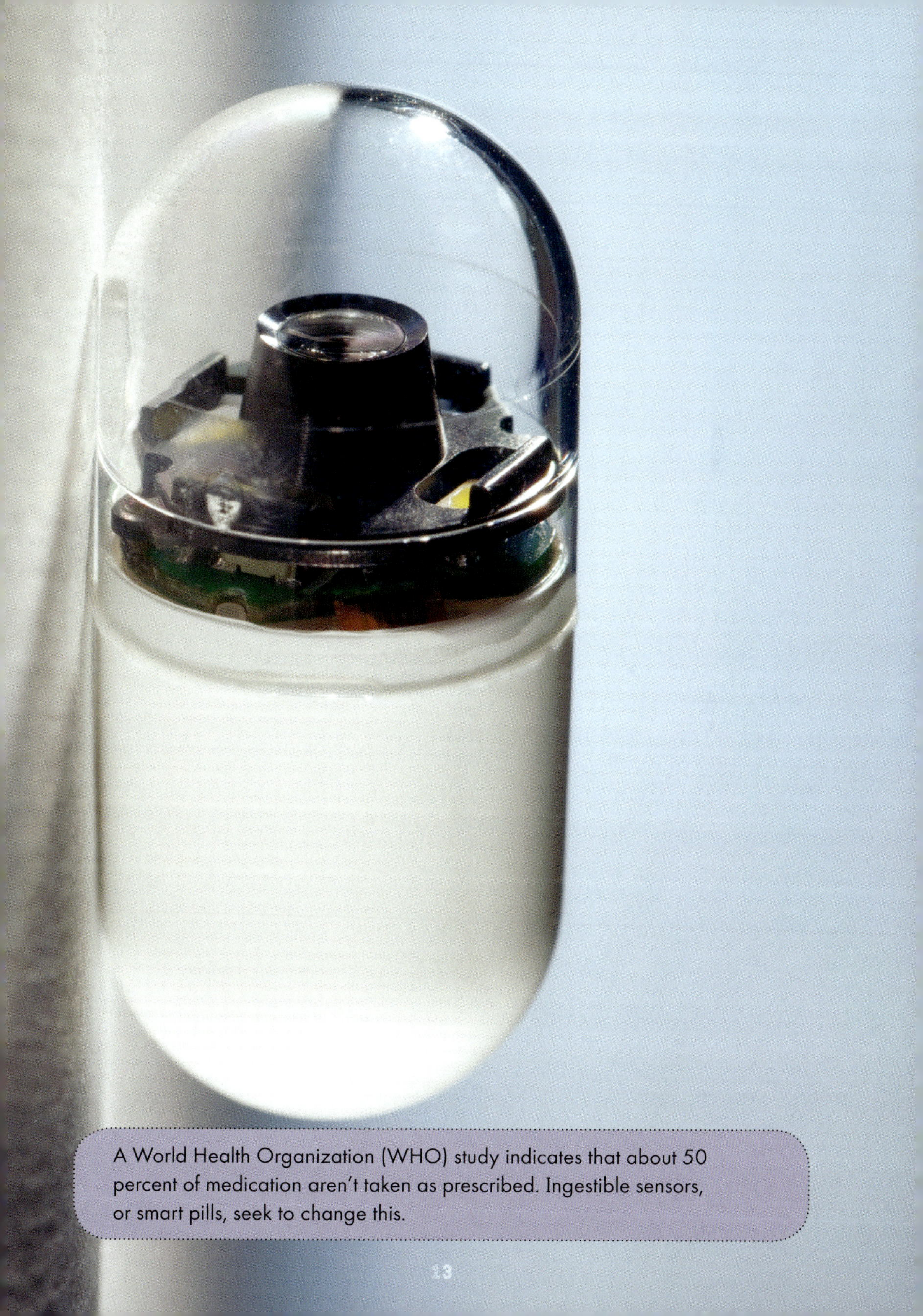

A World Health Organization (WHO) study indicates that about 50 percent of medication aren't taken as prescribed. Ingestible sensors, or smart pills, seek to change this.

CHAPTER TWO

Pros and Cons of Smart Healthcare

Healthcare is a complex process. About 15 million doctors care for billions of patients. There are more than 16,000 hospitals around the world. About one-third are in the United States. And health **insurance** companies must try to make care affordable.

The Internet of Things could impact everyone involved. The potential advantages to patients, doctors, and hospitals are enormous. That would mean far superior and cheaper healthcare. For instance, IoT-focused healthcare could potentially help decrease the cost of medical treatment, reduce medical errors, improve the patient-doctor relationship and experience, help patients and doctors better manage treatment plans, and so much more!

The general public got a head start on its benefits. Wearable devices like fitness and activity trackers monitor a wide range of health concerns. This helps people take **preventive** action.

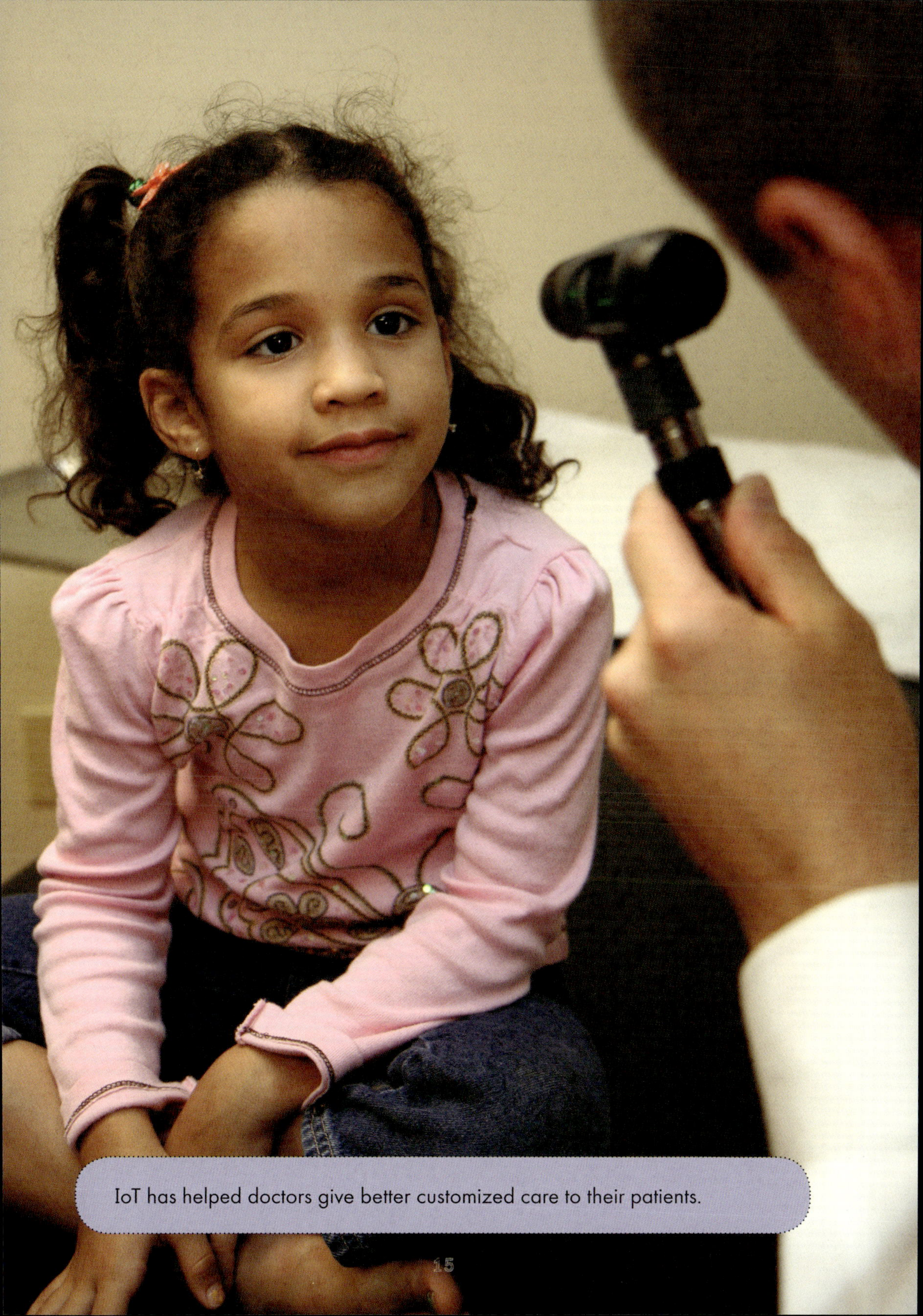

IoT has helped doctors give better customized care to their patients.

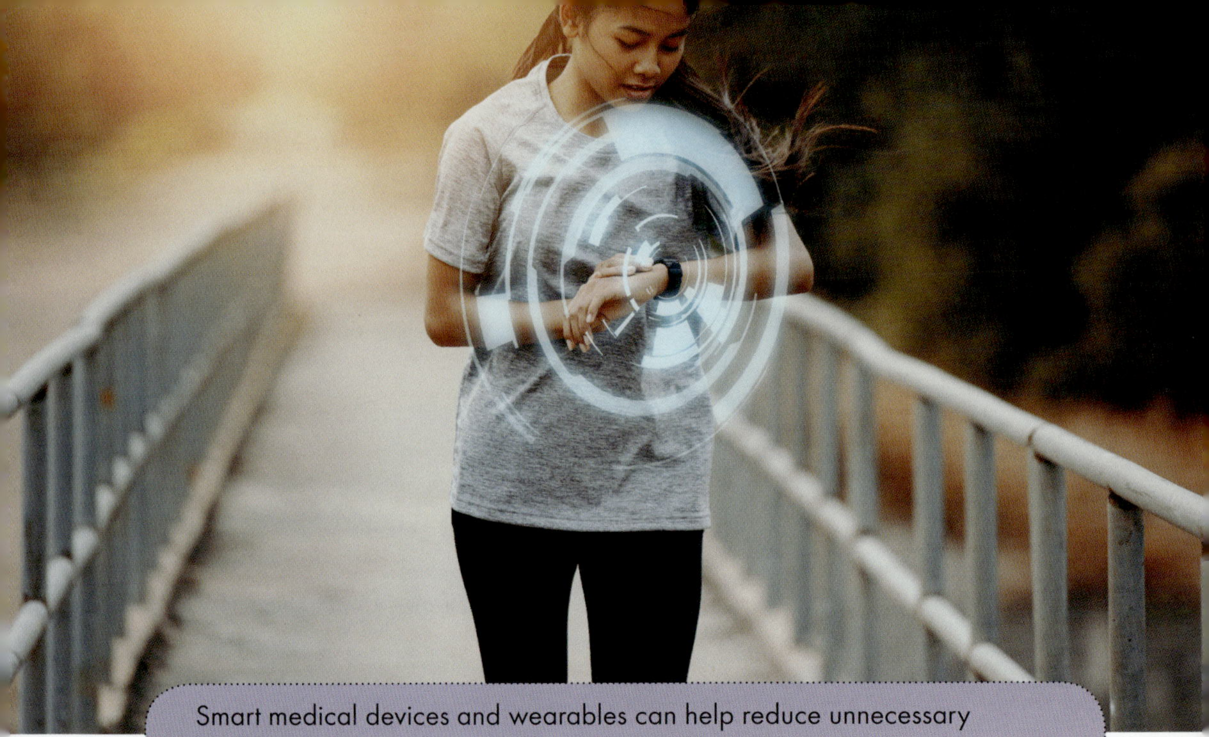

Smart medical devices and wearables can help reduce unnecessary doctor visits.

That data can also be presented to healthcare providers. Doctors have already benefited from IoT technology. They receive information sent by wearable sensors. They also check data received from sensors embedded in IoT home health monitors.

Doctors can create treatment plans based on that data. And they can do this without having to see the patient. This saves time for both the doctor and the patient. IoT technology can also save lives. The technology allows doctors to react to life-threatening problems in real time. They can send an ambulance immediately. Patients can get to hospitals faster.

Healthcare data can impact the insurance industry. According to the Centers for Medicare & Medicaid Services, national health spending is expected to reach $6 trillion by 2027.

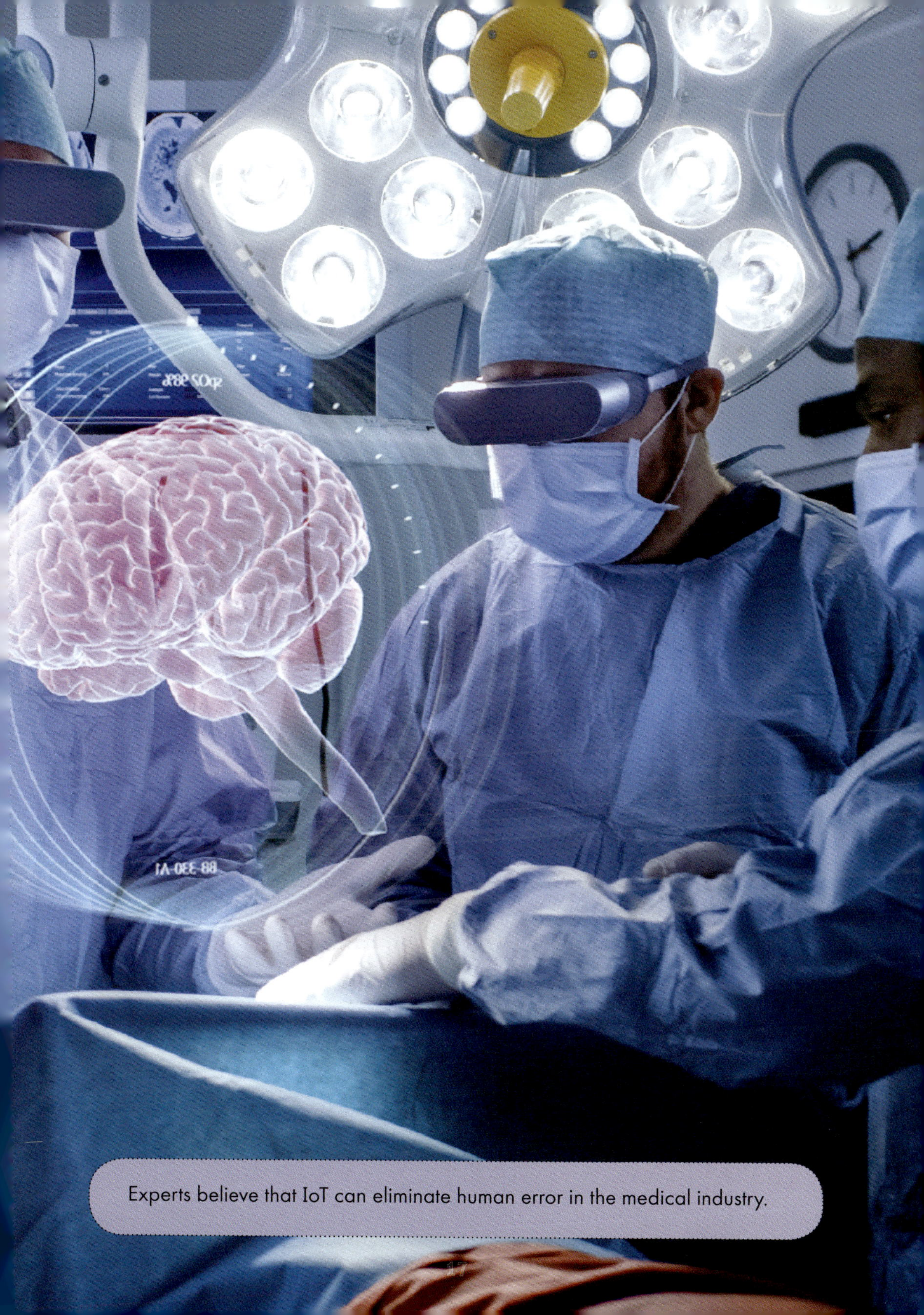

Experts believe that IoT can eliminate human error in the medical industry.

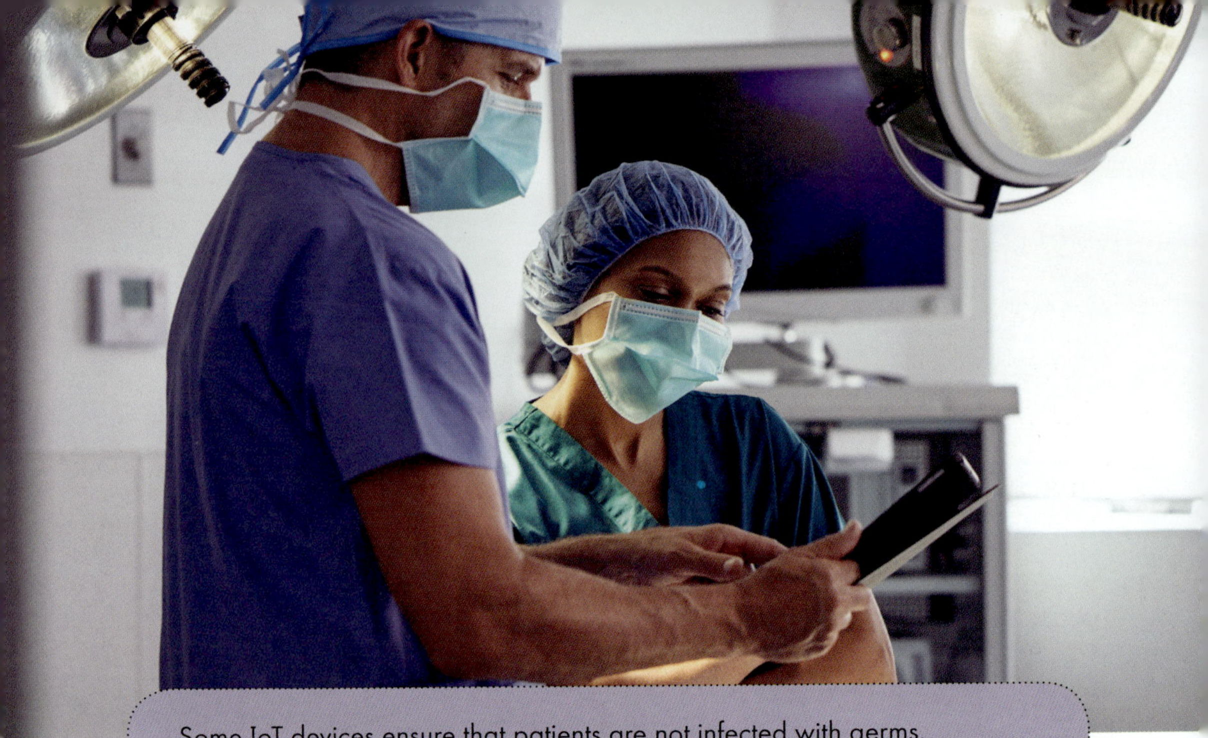

Some IoT devices ensure that patients are not infected with germs.

Since IoT data ensures accurate assessments, IoT technology could result in patients saving money.

The benefits of IoT in healthcare promise to outweigh the negatives. But there are concerns. Among them is privacy. Systems can get hacked and health information stolen. The need for security could raise costs. But the data is stored on a **cloud**-based system; the potential for hacks is always present. Altered data could cause doctors to change treatments based on wrong information. That could be dangerous. The hacked data could be sold to an outside party.

Security breaches are a significant danger. Limiting access of IoT devices to trusted healthcare personnel will be required.

Another concern is expense and **standardization**. It costs money for both the patient and the doctor to switch to IoT-focused healthcare. The patient may need to purchase or rent equipment, and the doctor or hospital may need to invest in IoT machines and systems. Standardization is important in healthcare. IoT-connected medical devices and systems can be accessed and operated from hospitals, clinics, and even patients' homes. Standards allow these devices and systems to operate together seamlessly. Standards also give doctors and patients peace of mind knowing that the data is recorded in the same manner across devices and systems.

STORY OF SURGICAL ROBOTS

Movies and television usually show robots with human qualities. They have arms, legs, and faces. They walk in human fashion. But in the real world, robots are machines that do simple or difficult tasks more easily than people. And IoT technology has helped to make them useful in hospitals. IoT-connected robots serve many purposes, including in surgery.

By 2017, smart robots had already assisted in some surgeries. They can be operated through smartphones. They are more flexible and precise in their movements than human **surgeons**. This allows them to complete more complex procedures. Robotic arms are considered especially helpful in joint replacement and spinal surgery.

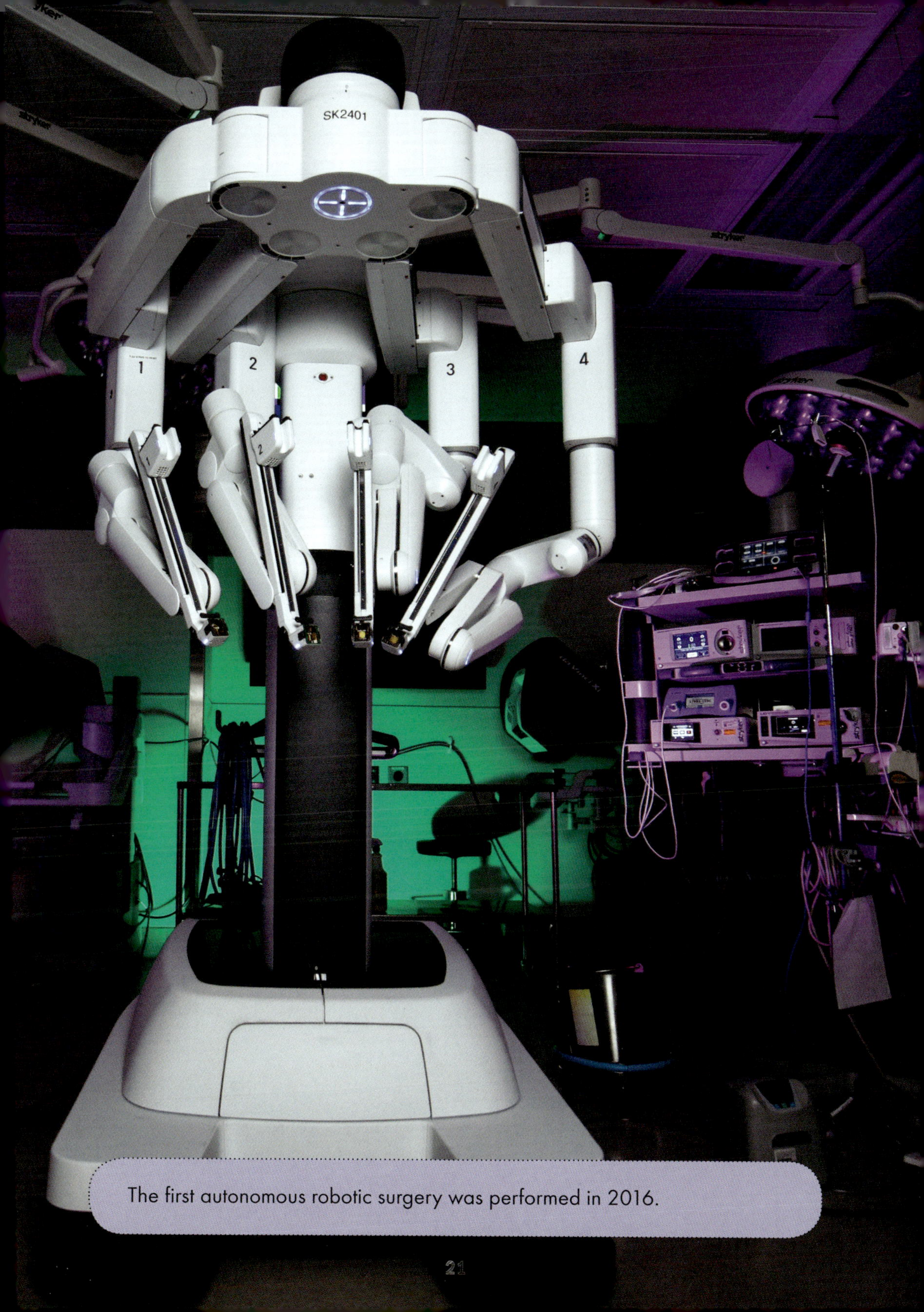

The first autonomous robotic surgery was performed in 2016.

CHAPTER THREE

The Future of IoT Healthcare

Healthcare is the most important target of IoT technology. It is where IoT has the greatest potential. Its ability to help people monitor their health became its first benefit to society. And its future is all about gaining acceptance and getting **implemented**. The increased use of fitness and activity trackers appears certain. Consumers also seem sure to use connected devices that alert family members and doctors to changes in condition.

But the Internet of Things promises far more. The technology will grow as a tool to discover new methods to prevent diseases. More doctors will use it to help diagnose and treat patients. IoT technology will be utilized to assist in surgery.

One study showed that 160 million IoT healthcare devices were expected to be in use by 2020. The result should be cheaper

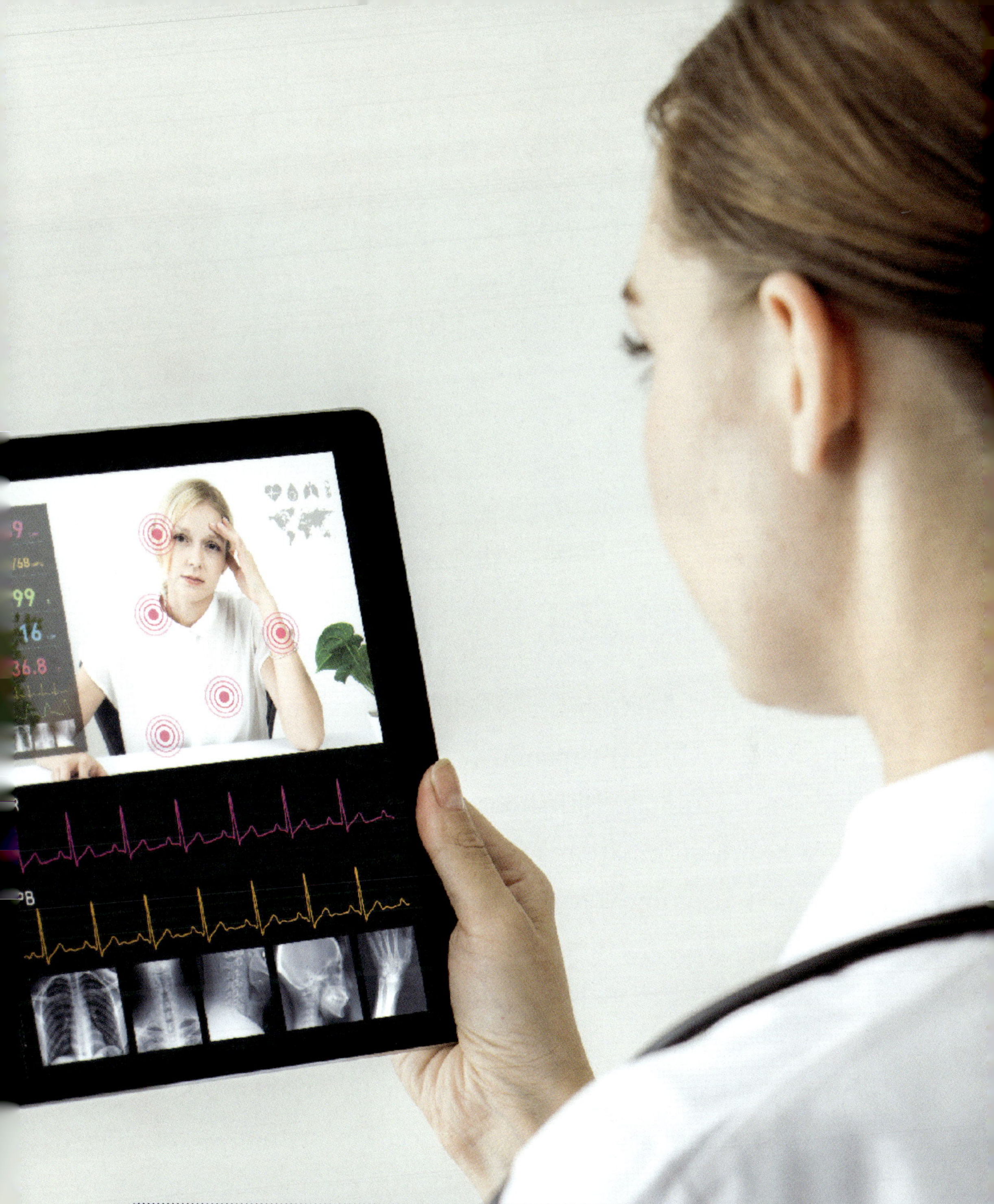

According to a study, there are about 40 doctors for every 100,000 people in rural areas in the United States. IoT can change this and help increase accessibility between patients and doctors.

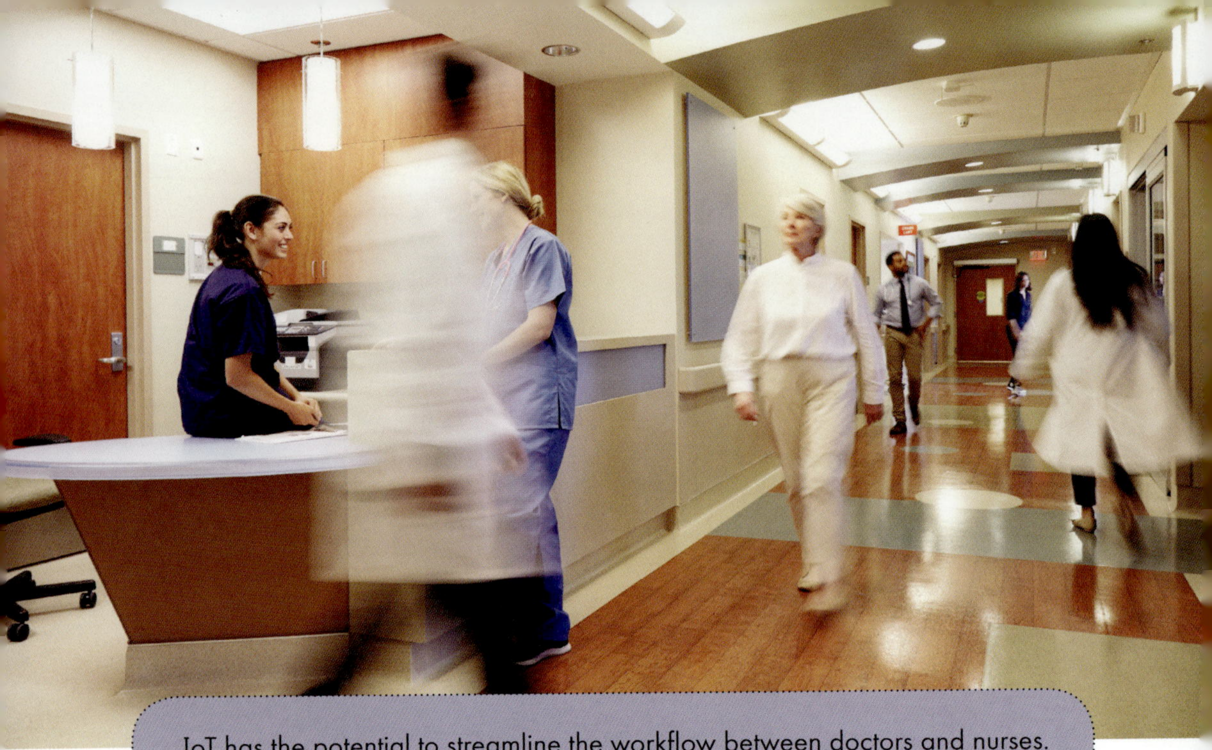

IoT has the potential to streamline the workflow between doctors and nurses.

and more efficient healthcare. Manufacturers will continue to create devices with IoT capability.

Another advantage is that doctors will have greater access to patient health information. Data from connected devices will be delivered in real time. That will allow doctors to prescribe treatment and medication faster. The accuracy of such data will help them make a more precise diagnosis.

The most critical result will be lives saved. IoT devices that send crucial data to doctors will speed up the entire process. They will have information to make decisions without seeing patients. Doctors can react immediately to emergencies such as heart attacks or strokes. Their advice to patients might prevent trips to the hospital. Or the device could send an ambulance to whisk them to the emergency room. Companies like Honeywell have created biometric devices that provide "an oximeter, blood pressure monitor and precision health scale" for patients.

IoT technology promises to make hospitals more efficient and productive. Connected devices will monitor the locations of doctors and nurses. They will be better able to communicate with each other. Another function of IoT that will positively impact hospitals is equipment monitoring. Sensors that detect flaws in critical devices will signal this to hospital personnel. The ability to stop breakdowns before they happen can save lives.

Many challenges await. Among them will be storing data from millions of IoT devices. Security concerns will result when the data is received and shared. Such concerns seem minor compared to the potential benefits of IoT in healthcare. A steady increase of IoT technology appears certain.

MANAGING MEDICATION THROUGH IOT

The task of keeping track of medication schedules can be overwhelming and confusing. People easily forget if they have taken their pills. Or they forget to take them at all. Studies estimate that patients failing to take their pills affects not only them—it also results in about 10 percent of all hospital visits! This costs the American healthcare system nearly $300 billion a year. IoT technology has a solution with smart wireless pill bottles that track medication schedules.

One such product is Pillsy. It is enabled by Bluetooth. The device knows when people open and close the cap, and determines if they have taken their medication. It pairs with an app that reminds people when to take a pill. It can even follow up with a text or phone call.

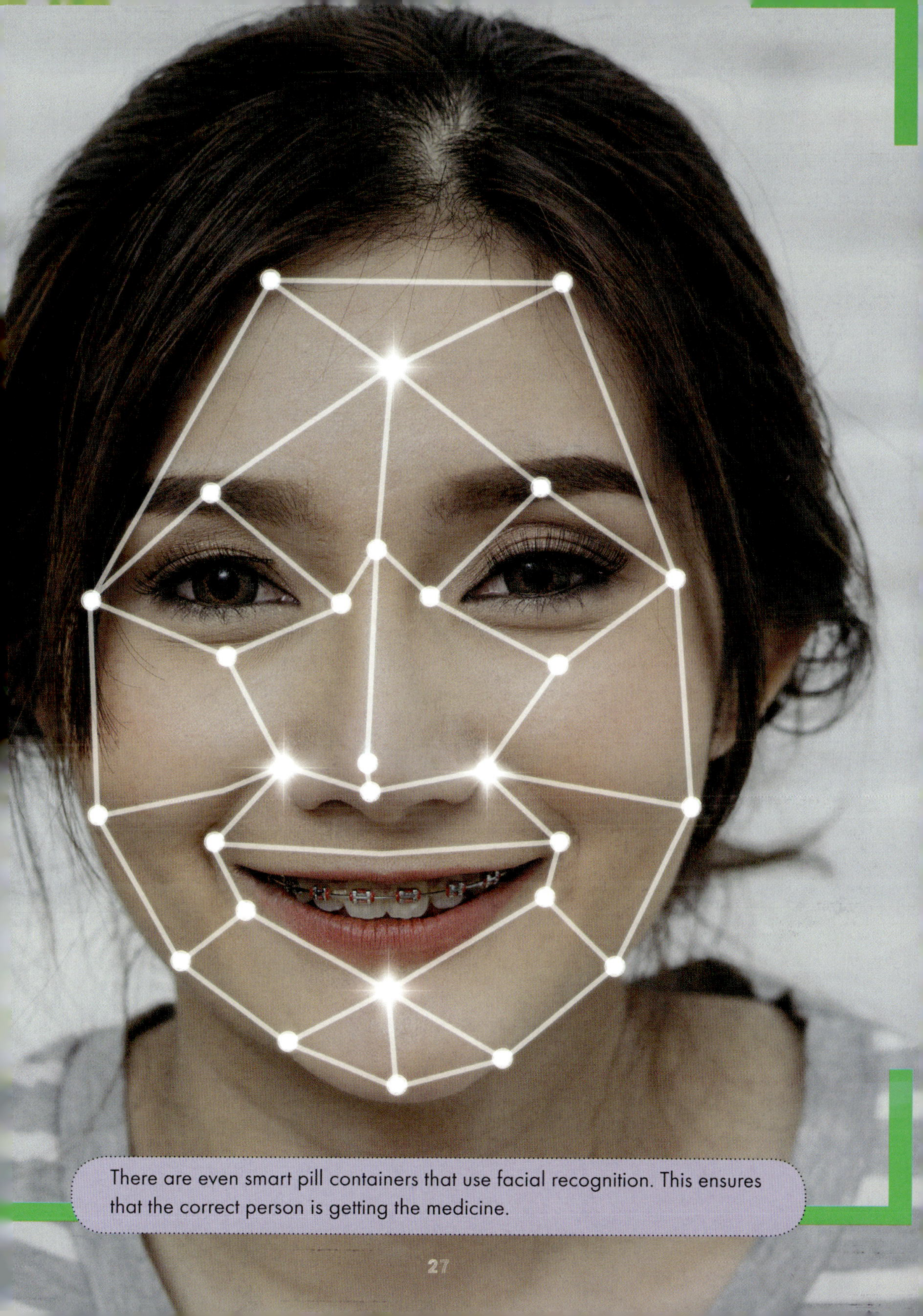

There are even smart pill containers that use facial recognition. This ensures that the correct person is getting the medicine.

Collaboration

Healthcare is critical to everyone. The Internet of Things could help all involved in the process. Security issues can't be allowed to halt the progress of IoT technology.

People have used IoT to monitor many aspects of their health on their own. The ability to know the warning signs of an emergency is a crucial benefit of that technology. It must not be compromised. Only those in the medical field who can be trusted should have access to personal information. But hospitals and other medical centers must decide who can be trusted. They have to arrive at a fair decision process.

Think About It

How should people in the medical world decide who, aside from patients' personal doctors, can have access to IoT healthcare data?

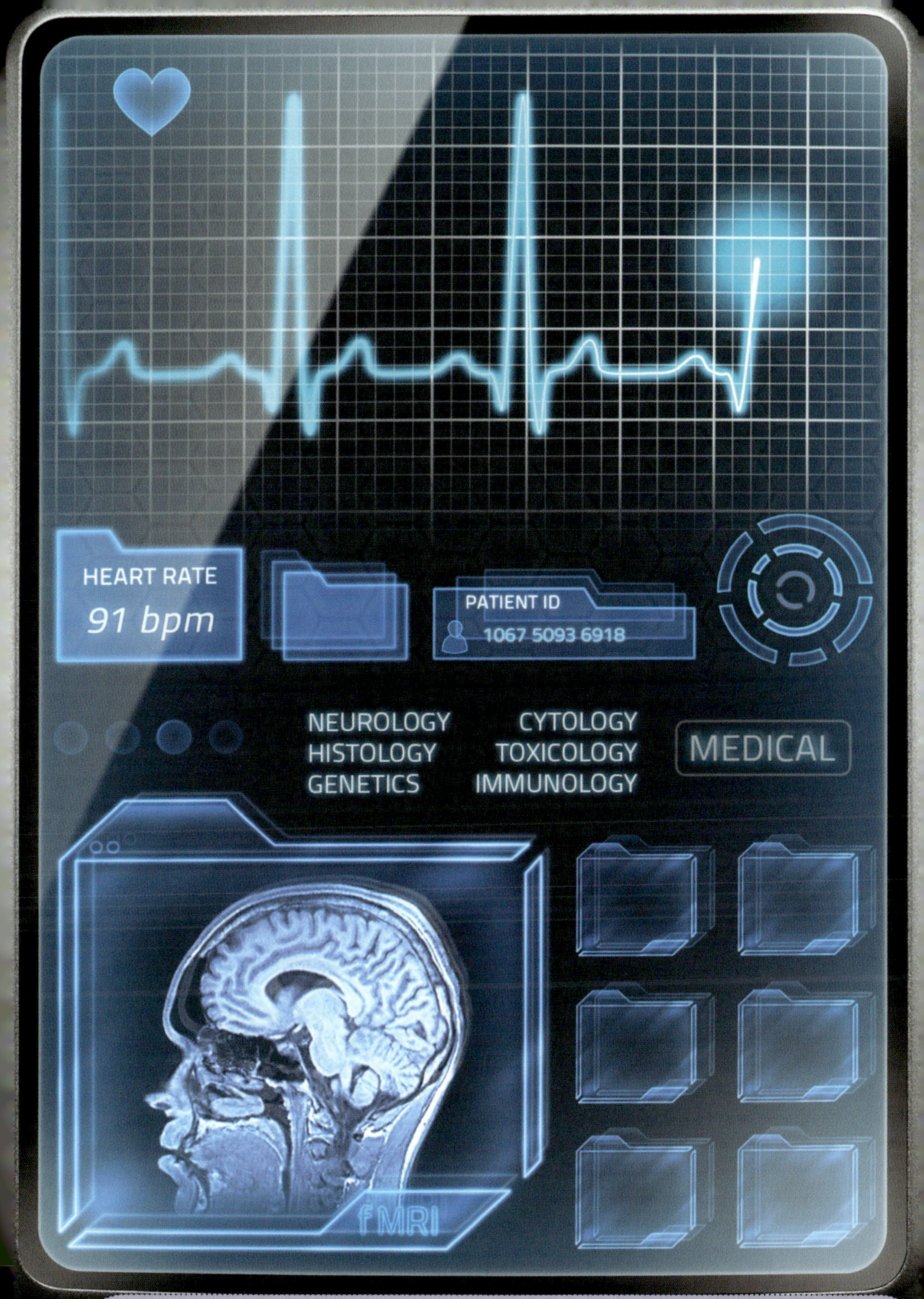

The healthcare industry is going through a digital transformation, all thanks to the Internet of Things.

Learn More

Books

Fritz, Zoe, and Katie Daynes. *Look Inside a Hospital*. London, England: Usborne Publishing, 2018.

Stevenson, Tyler. *Health Care: Limits, Laws, and Lives at Stake*. New York, NY: Lucent Press, 2019.

Todaro, Joseph. *Blockchain*. Ann Arbor, MI: Cherry Lake Publishing, 2020.

Websites

Kinooze: The Internet of Things
http://kinooze.com/the-internet-of-things
Learn more about what IoT devices can do.

YouTube—Aruba: The Rise of IoT in Healthcare
https://www.youtube.com/watch?v=Y8288eEEsmc
Discover how IoT can potentially save lives.

Glossary

allergens (AL-ur-jenz) substances that can cause an allergic reaction

asthma (AZ-muh) lung disease that makes it difficult to breathe

cataracts (KAT-uh-rakts) a clouding of the eye lens that makes it difficult to see

cloud (KLOUD) network of remote servers around the world

cognitive (KAHG-nih-tiv) use of the mind to gain knowledge

data (DAY-tuh) facts to be used for planning or making decisions

diagnose (dye-uhg-NOHS) to figure out a physical or mental problem based on examination

gastroparesis (gas-trow-PAH-ree-sehs) a medical condition in which the stomach is unable to function correctly

implemented (IM-pluh-ment-id) put into place

influx (IN-fluks) the arrival of a large amount of something

insulin (IN-suh-lin) hormone in the pancreas that controls and regulates the body's use of sugars

insurance (in-SHOOR-uhns) an arrangement in which a patient pays money to a company that agrees to pay for certain costs that cover an illness

monitored (MAH-nih-turd) checked on or kept track of something

prescribe (prih-SKRIBE) to write an order for a specific kind of medicine for a patient

preventive (prih-VEN-tiv) measures taken to prevent a negative outcome

sensors (SEN-surz) detection devices that respond by transmitting a signal

standardization (stan-dur-dih-ZAY-shuhn) the changing of things so they are similar and consistent

surgeons (SUR-juhnz) doctors who perform operations on patients

symptoms (SIMP-tuhmz) signs of a physical illness or disease

Index